Ketogenic Diet

Ketosis: Recipes for Every Taste to Burn Body Fat and Lose Weight Fast

Contents

information is without contract or any type of guarantee assurance.

The trademarks that are used are without any consent, and the publication of the trademark is without permission or backing by the trademark owner. All trademarks and brands within this book are for clarifying purposes only and are the owned by the owners themselves, not affiliated with this document.

Introduction

I want to thank you and commend you for purchasing the book, **"Ketosis: *Ketogenic Diet Recipes for Every Taste to Burn Body Fat and Lose Weight Fast"*.**

This book contains everything you need to know about the ketogenic diet and why it's so effective for weight loss. More importantly, in these pages, you'll find 50 mouthwatering recipes that will enable you to obtain your ultimate fitness goal.

The key to a successful weight loss plan is simple: commitment. The primary reason why so many weight watchers find it difficult to commit to their routine is because the weight loss plan is unsustainable. The inessential deprivation, which is an inevitable part of most weight loss diets, only tempts you to cheat. Thus, instigating your downward spiral towards unwholesome eating habits.

Moreover, with unattainable ingredients and inconvenient preparation techniques, most weight loss plans are doomed to fail right from the start. What you need is a diet plan that you can easily fit into your daily lifestyle. No weird ingredients. No need to slave away in the kitchen for hours and hours. And absolutely no need to slink away from your friends, family, and colleagues during mealtimes.

You are the product of what you feed yourself on a regular basis. In this book, you'll find great recipes that will take you through breakfast, lunch, dinner, and even those moments in between. These meals are delicious, satiating, healthy, natural and easy to prepare. They are the fruits of meticulous research, epicurean experimentations, and a real passion for achieving wellness.

Read on and you'll discover what the ketogenic diet is all about: *Real* food for *real* individuals with *real* lives who want *real results*!

Thanks again for purchasing this book, I hope you enjoy it!

Chapter 1:
Beginning Your Journey to Fitness

What is the Ketogenic Diet? Why is it effective?

The Keto diet is a weight loss diet that promotes the consumption of high-fat edibles while minimizing or totally eliminating the intake of carbohydrates. Ketogenic dieters are encouraged to consume moderate amounts of protein-rich food.

The Keto diet's ultimate goal is to help your body reach a ketotic state. When your body is in ketosis, it uses fat as fuel in lieu of carbohydrates. Fat becomes the body's chief energy source for carrying out its daily functions. Thus, you end up burning fat deposits in place of glucose. Once your body gets used to a ketotic state, this results to weight loss which is natural and long-lasting.

How safe is ketosis?

Very. In fact, you may not know it but your body naturally reverts to a state of ketosis each time you fast or miss a meal. This is a safe and natural survival mechanism of the human body, which enabled our predecessors from the hunter and gatherer era to live through winter and food scarcity. Every time you ingest a meal that's high in fat, low in carbs, and with moderate protein, the body is prompted to undergo a ketotic state.

Isn't a high fat diet dangerous?

When following the ketogenic diet, you are encouraged to consume *good* fats. These consist of oils which are unrefined and rich in Omega-3.

Is it possible for the body to survive without carbohydrates?

Yes. This is evidenced by ethnic groups such as the Masai of East Africa, the Inuit of the Canadian Arctic, and the Chukotka of Russia. All of these groups do not include carbohydrate-rich food sources in their diet.

What you need to understand is that your liver is capable of making all the glucose that your brain requires in order to function. The human body creates its own glucose using non-carbohydrate carbon substrates. This is called gluconeogenesis. All you need to do is to alter your diet so that your body will eventually grow used to utilizing and burning fat for fuel.

That said, you don't really need to completely eliminate carbs from your meals. You only need to ensure that you consume 20-60 grams of carbs daily. The source of your carbs must be from vegetables, raw dairy products, nuts, and fruits which are low in carbohydrates. In other words, only up to 10% of your daily calories should be from carbohydrates. Up to 20% of your daily calories should be from protein-rich sources. All the rest should be from fats (70% or more).

Diet Don't:

One common error that dieters make is to mistake the ketogenic diet for a high-protein diet. If you end up consuming too much protein, this places you at risk for developing "rabbit starvation". This condition is characterized by persistent cravings that will cause you to eat more than what's recommended.

Begin the Journey

- You start your journey to weight loss and wellness by checking your pantry. Remove all carb-rich edibles.

- Next, replace all the food you've lost with items which are rich in good fat and low in carbohydrates.

- When shopping for food, opt for organic, non-processed varieties.

- Scrutinize the labels, specifically the carb count. When buying meat products, make sure that each pack has no more than 2 g of carbs. Each pack of vegetables should have no more than 5 g of carbohydrates. Just because a product is advertised as low carb, that doesn't mean that it is. Beware of "hidden" carbohydrates which are usually contained in food additives in frozen goods and "sugar-free" items.

- Instead of eating three main meals, begin with small frequent ones.

- Monitor your progress by using a blood ketone meter. You'll know you've reached a keto-adapted state when your serum ketones are at a minimum of 0.5 mM to a maximum of 3.0 mM. Alternatively, you may use OTC urine strips. When using the latter, be sure to test before going to bed because ketone concentrations peak at night.

- To combat the side effects of the ketogenic diet such as dizziness, constipation, dehydration, and fruity breath, make sure that you drink lots of water.

Diet Don't:

Just because you're dieting that doesn't mean you should skip physical exercise entirely. Avoid leading a sedentary lifestyle. You don't have to develop a strenuous workout routine. In fact, heavy exercise is discouraged because it might cause you to crave carbs in between activities. Instead, engage in mild aerobic exercises.

Which foods are safe to eat?

- Meat is certainly allowed. This can be of the fresh or frozen variety. Don't think that your options are limited to beef, chicken, and pork. Explore other sources like lamb, venison, pheasant, duck meat, goat, etc. Organ meats are highly nutritious. Just make sure that your sources are organic and grass-fed. You can do a lot of things with meat from roasting and grilling to frying and sautéing. Contrary to what you might think, the ketogenic diet doesn't encourage you to eat all the meat that you want. Instead, you are advised to enjoy food only until you reach a satiety point.

- When it comes to fish, the wild-caught variety is recommended. Examples are salmon, cod, and halibut. Shellfish like lobsters, scallops, and shrimp may also be included in your diet.

- Hard-boiled eggs are safe and quick emergency snacks for ketogenic dieters. In fact, a lot of the recipes you'll find in this book use eggs as an ingredient. Ensure that the eggs you use are fresh and free-range.

- Your chief source of fiber should be from green leafy vegetables. Consider spinach, kale, lettuce, and other leafy greens as kitchen staples. Nightshades, sea vegetables, and cruciferous vegetables like eggplant, nori, and cauliflowers are to be eaten in moderation. The same rule applies to sprouts and okra. As for sweet potatoes and other root vegetables, you may enjoy them infrequently.

- Fatty fruits like avocadoes and coconuts are recommended. Low-carb berries are to be consumed in moderation. There are also some fruits which must only be taken on occasion and these include peaches, apricots, and watermelons. You may snack on dried fruits like raisins but eat them in small amounts.

- Other recommended snacks include almonds, macadamias, pumpkin seeds, watermelon seeds, pecans, and hazelnuts. However, there are also nuts which must only be eaten occasionally. These include cashews and pistachios.

- Decaf coffee and tea are allowed. So are unsweetened wines. However, you are advised to imbibe only on rare occasions. As far as the keto diet is concerned, water will always be the best beverage.

Diet Don't:

During the first few weeks, it would be best to keep away from starchy vegetables like carrots, squash, and zucchini. Otherwise, you'll be pulled out of your ketotic state. Afterwards, you may gradually reintroduce them to your diet. They make great substitutes for the carbs that you're missing.

More Tips:

- When frying, substitute breading mix with pork cracklings.

- Make your own condiments, from ketchup to mustard to mayo. Ferment kimchi and kombucha at home. Remember that no food company will ever care for your health as much as you do, so homemade anything is preferable to grocery items. However, if this isn't possible, then opt for brands that contain the least amount of carbs.

- As much as possible, improve your dishes with fresh herbs instead of store-bought flavorings.

- In place of sugar, use carb-free sweeteners such as stevia.

- You may add whey protein into your diet plan. Just be sure that you screen it for carb-rich additives and synthetic sweeteners.

- To thicken soups, you may use arrowroot powder in reasonable amounts.

- The great thing about the ketogenic diet is that you don't have to say goodbye to chocolate. Use cocoa and carob powder in baking and cooking. However, when buying extra dark chocolate, it should be 70% or more.

Chapter 2:
Healthy Mornings and New Beginnings

1) Not So Classic Bacon and Eggs

6 eggs, free-range, hard-boiled and peeled

12 strips bacon, organic

3.5 oz. organic cream cheese, full-fat

¼ tsp. dehydrated thyme

- First, warm up the oven to 400 F.

- To make the cream cheese filling, use a spoon to mix the cream cheese and the dried thyme.

- Slice the eggs lengthways. Carefully scoop out the yolks. Eat or keep the yolks for other recipes.

- Spoon some of the cream cheese filling into the egg hollows. Fill six halves and then cover with the other six halves.

- Fry the bacon. Place on a plate with paper towels. Leave to cool to room temperature.

- Next, wrap each egg with a couple of bacon strips.

- Arrange the bacon-wrapped eggs on a glass baking tray.

- Cook in the oven for half an hour.

- Enjoy!

2) Keto Cream Cheese Pancakes

2 eggs, free-range

2 oz. organic cream cheese, full-fat

1 tsp. sucralose-based sugar alternative

½ tsp. cinnamon

- Place all the ingredients together in a blender.

- Blend until you obtain a smooth consistency.

- Leave for a couple of minutes to allow the bubbles to settle.

- Grease a skillet with some organic butter.

- Then, pour ¼ of the batter into it.

- Cook for a couple of minutes or until you get a nice golden hue.

- Flip and then cook for another full minute.

- Dig in!

Note: This recipe is good for 4.

3) Ketogenic Cajun Hash

1 tbsp. ghee

453 g cauliflower

226 g pastrami, shaved

½ white onion

½ green bell pepper

2 tbsp. garlic, minced

1 tsp. Cajun seasoning

- Steam the cauliflower.

- Meanwhile, prepare the vegetables. Cut up the onion into ¼ inch slices. Then, cut up the bell pepper to ¼ inch slices.

- Slice the pastrami to 1 inch pieces.

- When the cauliflower is ready, slice into tiny chunks. Squeeze out the extra water.

- Adjust the stove's setting to medium heat.

- Heat the ghee in a skillet and then sauté the onions for approximately five minutes.

- Throw in the garlic and cook for another couple of minutes.

- Next, add the cauliflower. Cook for about seven minutes or until it becomes crispy.

- With continuous mixing, sprinkle with Cajun seasoning.

- Afterwards, throw in the pastrami.

- Add the bell pepper.

- Continue cooking for 5 more minutes.

- Then, distribute the Cajun hash into serving bowls.

- Top with eggs cooked sunny side up if you wish.

4) Keto Skillet Baked Eggs

4 eggs, free-range

5 oz. plain yogurt, full-fat

10 oz. spinach

2 tbsp. butter, organic and unsalted

1 clove garlic, cut to half

2 1/2 tbsp. leek, chopped (just the white parts)

2 1/2 tbsp. green onion (just the light green and white parts)

2 tbsp. coconut oil

1 tsp. lemon juice

1 tsp. oregano, chopped

¼ tsp. red pepper flakes

Sea salt (desired amount)

A pinch of paprika

- Warm up the oven to 300 F.

- In a bowl, combine the yogurt and the garlic. Add some sea salt. Mix well.

- Adjust the stove's setting to medium heat.

- In a pan, melt half of the butter.

- Then, adjust the stove's setting to low. Cook the green onion and the leek for approximately 10 minutes.

- Throw in the spinach.

- Add the lemon juice.

- Sprinkle with desired amount of salt.

- Adjust the stove's setting to medium high and cook for 5 more minutes.

- Next, pour the mixture into a baking dish. Be sure not to include any extra fluid.

- At the middle of the spinach, create 4 deep depressions.

- Afterwards, break an egg into each indentation.

- Place the dish in the oven and cook for about 12-13 minutes.

- Adjust the stove's setting to medium-low. Then, melt the remaining butter in a saucepan.

- Throw in the pepper flakes, the paprika, and some sea salt. Cook for a couple of minutes. Sprinkle with oregano and cook for an extra one half minute.

- Scoop out the garlic from the yogurt.

- Then, slather the yogurt over the eggs and spinach.

- Grab two forks and share with someone special.

Note: This recipe is good for two.

5) Keto Cinnamon "Oatmeal"

4 oz. hot water

64 g golden flax meal

64 g desiccated coconut, unsweetened

2 tbsp. coconut milk

64 g chia seeds

1 tsp. cinnamon powder

Raw wild honey

- In a bowl, mix the golden flax meal, the chia seeds, and the desiccated coconut. Sprinkle cinnamon and combine thoroughly.

- Transfer the mixture into an air-tight glass jar.

- Then, take 64 g of the mixture and pour it into a bowl.

- Pour 4 oz. hot water over it. Cover and leave for about 4 minutes.

- Stir in the coconut milk.

- Sweeten with raw wild honey.

- Use blueberries or raspberries as toppings if you wish.

- Enjoy your breakfast!

6) Keto Egg Puffs

32 g Pecorino Romano cheese, grated

4 eggs, free-range

32 g chives, chopped

32 g bacon bits

Freshly ground black pepper

- Separate the egg yolks from the eggs whites. All of the egg whites should be in one bowl. Meanwhile, each yolk must be in an individual bowl.

- Beat the egg whites to create stiff peaks.

- With continuous and gentle beating, add the Pecorino Romano and the bacon bits.

- While still mixing, throw in the chives.

- Preheat the oven to 450 F.

- Line a baking dish with parchment paper.

- Scoop the mixture into the dish to make four mounds.

- Create a depression into the middle of each mound.

- Place the dish in the oven and cook for approximately 3 minutes.

- Afterwards, carefully spoon each egg yolk into each hollow.

- Sprinkle with desired amount of black pepper.

- Bake for another couple of minutes.

7) Keto Breakfast Egg Muffins

3 eggs, free-range

453 g. mild sausage

36 oz. leafy greens, chopped (ex. Swiss chards)

2 oz. parmesan, shredded

64 g onion, chopped

1 tsp. coconut oil

16 oz. ricotta cheese (whole milk variety)

1 garlic clove, finely chopped

1/8 tsp. nutmeg powder

8 oz. mozzarella, shredded

Sea salt

Freshly ground black pepper

- Preheat the oven to 350 F.

- Meanwhile, heat the coconut oil in a skillet. Then, sauté the garlic and onions until the latter is softened.

- Next, add the greens. Cook for approximately 5 minutes.

- Sprinkle with sea salt, black pepper, and nutmeg powder.

- Turn off the stove and leave to cool.

- In a big bowl, whisk the eggs.

- Gradually fold in the three cheeses.

- Then, add the sautéed greens. Mix well.

- Line the muffin tins with sausage. Press ¼ inch thick sausage into each cup.

- Afterwards, scoop some of the mixture into each muffin cup until each cup is ¾ full.

- Arrange the tins on a baking sheet lined with parchment paper. Place in the oven and bake for half an hour.

- Enjoy the first meal of the day with loved ones!

Note: This recipe makes 12 muffins.

8) Keto Breakfast Pizza

2 eggs, free-range

6 slices pepperoni

1 oz. mozzarella, diced

5 pcs. small tomatoes, sliced

2 tsp. coconut oil

7 pcs. black olives, sliced

¼ tsp. dehydrated oregano

Freshly ground black pepper

Sea salt

- Warm up the oven toaster.

- Beat the eggs.

- Cut up the pepperoni slices into halves.

- Adjust the stove's setting to medium heat.

- Place coconut oil in a skillet and heat for about 60 seconds.

- Then, add the eggs. Sprinkle with salt and pepper.

- Add dried oregano.

- Cook the eggs for a couple of minutes.

- Next, arrange half of the tomatoes on the eggs.

- Layer with half of the pepperoni.

- Arrange half of the olives on the pepperoni.

- Add half of the diced mozzarella on top of the pepperoni.

- Repeat layering until all ingredients are used up.

- Place a lid on the skillet and cook for about three minutes.

- Afterwards, cook in an oven toaster for another 5 minutes.

- Enjoy it while it's hot.

9) Green Breakfast Shake

½ avocado, sliced to small chunks

10 oz. almond milk, unsweetened

1 tsp. matcha

2 oz. vanilla whey protein powder

4 oz. plain yogurt

1 tbsp. hot water

2 tsp. erythritol

- Melt the matcha in hot water.

- Combine all the ingredients in a blender.

- Then, blend until you get a smooth texture.

- Pour into two tall serving glasses.

- Drink up!

10) Choco-Hazelnut Granola

192 g hazelnuts

2 oz. hazelnut oil

½ tsp. hazelnut essence

32 g raw cocoa powder, unsweetened

2 oz. chocolate, unsweetened

128 g flax seed meal

2 oz. organic butter, melted

192 g almonds

67 g erythritol

½ tsp. sea salt

20 drops liquid stevia

- First, warm up the oven to 300 F.

- Use parchment paper to line a baking dish.

- Combine the almonds and the hazelnuts in a food processor. Pulse until you get rough crumbs.

- Pour into a bowl and mix with flax seed meal.

- Add sea salt and cocoa powder. Mix thoroughly.

- Adjust the stove's setting to low.

- Melt the butter in a saucepan. Add the chocolate and the hazelnut oil with continuous stirring.

- Still stirring, add the erythritol.

- Then, take the pan away from heat.

- Add the hazelnuts and instill the drops of stevia. Mix well.

- With constant stirring, gradually pour the chocolate mixture into the nut mixture.

- Transfer the mix into the baking dish.

- Place in the oven. Baking time is approximately 15 minutes. However, be sure to stir the mixture every five minutes.

- After the granola is done, leave it to sit in the oven for half an hour or less.

Note: This recipe makes 10 servings.

11) Small Salmon Frittatas

6 whole eggs, free-range

8 egg whites

4 oz. smoked salmon, divided to ¼ inch slices

3 tbsp. full-fat milk

3 oz. organic cream cheese, cubed

1 tbsp. extra virgin coconut oil

32 g white onion, diced

2 tbsp. green onion, sliced thinly

½ tsp. sea salt

1/8 tsp. black pepper

- Heat up the oven to 325 F.

- Prepare six 8 oz. ramekins by coating them with cooking spray.

- Heat the coconut oil in a non-stick pan.

- Sauté the white onion for a couple of minutes.

- Sprinkle with desired amount of salt and pepper.

- Then, add the salmon. Stir for a few seconds.

- Remove from heat and leave to cool.

- In a bowl, mix the milk, the cream cheese, and the eggs.

- Scoop 2 tbsp. of the salmon mixture into each baking bowl.

- Then, pour 5 oz. of the egg mixture into each bowl.

- Arrange the baking bowls on a baking sheet.

- Place in the oven. Baking time is between 23-26 minutes.

- You'll know it's ready if you insert a toothpick into the frittata and it comes out neatly.

- Use the green onion for garnishing.

12) Keto Breakfast Bowl

4 eggs, free-range

128 g quinoa, cooked

6 oz. smoked salmon

1 avocado, sliced

2 tbsp. grape seed oil

Juice from ½ - 1 lemon

Green onion, chopped

¼ tsp. sea salt

¼ tsp. black pepper, freshly ground

- Adjust the stove's setting to medium heat.

- Cook the eggs with the skillet's lid on for about 3 minutes. This way, you'll get yolks that are somewhat runny.

- Sprinkle with sea salt and pepper.

- Lay the eggs on top of the quinoa.

- Arrange the salmon on top of the eggs.

- Then, arrange the avocado slices around the salmon.

- Squeeze desired amount of lemon juice.

- Lastly, use the green onion for garnishing.

- Bon appétit!

Chapter 3:
A Good Gastronomer's
Guide to Lunch

13) Rosemary Apple Chops

4 pcs. pork chops, organic

½ fresh apple, sliced

2 tbsp. coconut oil

2 tbsp. olive oil

2 tbsp. organic apple cider vinegar

4 rosemary sprigs

Juice from ½ lemon

1 tbsp. maple syrup, sugar-free

Sea salt

Freshly ground black pepper

Paprika (desired amount)

- In the oven, preheat the iron skillet to 400 F.

- Meanwhile, use paper towels to pat the meat dry.

- Rub coconut oil all over the meat.

- Rub desired amount of salt, paprika, and pepper on both sides.

- Adjust the stove's setting to high heat.

- Remove the skillet from the oven and place on the stove.

- For a couple of minutes, sear each side of the chops.

- Afterwards, arrange the apple slices on top of the meat.

- Put rosemary sprigs on top.

- Place the skillet in the oven and cook for approximately 10 minutes.

- Meanwhile, combine the lemon and the apple cider vinegar in a small bowl. Add desired amount of salt and pepper.

- Lastly, add the olive oil gradually with thorough whisking.

- When the chops are ready, drizzle the mixture all over the meat.

- Serve.

14) Keto Tiny Tuna Melts

10 oz. boiled tuna, drained and sliced to chunks

1 avocado, sliced to cubes

2 oz. homemade mayonnaise

45 g almond flour

2 oz. parmesan

4 oz. coconut oil

1 tsp. garlic, minced

½ tsp. shallots, minced

Sea salt

Freshly ground black pepper

- Place the tuna in a large bowl.

- Combine with mayonnaise.

- Mix in the parmesan cheese.

- With continuous tossing, add the spices.

- Throw in the avocado cubes. Mix but be careful not to mash it.

- Scatter the almond flour on a clean flat surface.

- With your hands, create small balls with the tuna mixture.

- Then, roll the balls in almond flour.

- Adjust the stove's setting to medium and heat the coconut oil.

- Afterwards, fry the tuna balls until you get a nice crispy texture.

- Remove from stovetop and transfer to a serving dish.

15) Keto Shrimp Spinach

36 oz. spinach

40 pcs shrimp, peeled

4 tbsp. organic butter

2 tbsp. coconut cream

2 tbsp. olive oil

½ white onion, finely chopped

6 garlic cloves, squeezed

1 tbsp. parmesan

- Heat the oil in a skillet.
- Cook the shrimp for a couple of minutes just until you get a pink hue.
- Remove from pan and set aside.
- Place the onion into the pan. Add a pinch of sea salt and cook until transparent.
- Add the garlic juice and cook for about 60 seconds.
- Next, add the coconut cream. Then, throw in the butter.
- Stir in the parmesan.
- Cook together for a couple of minutes to create a sauce.
- Afterwards, place the shrimp into the skillet.

- Cook with continuous stirring for about 2 ½ minutes.

- Make sure that the shrimp is completely covered with the sauce.

- After that, remove the shrimp from the pan.

- Now it's time to cook the spinach in the same skillet. Cook as desired. However, it's recommended that you cook the spinach only for a few seconds. The rawer, the better.

- Arrange the spinach on a serving platter.

- Then, arrange the shrimp on top of the spinach.

- Enjoy lunching with your loved ones!

Note: This recipe serves 4.

16) Quick Egg Drop Soup

2 eggs, free-range

12 oz. organic chicken broth

1 tbsp. organic butter

1 tsp. garlic, minced

½ cube chicken bouillon

- Adjust the stove's setting to medium-high.

- Then, combine the chicken broth, the cube, and the butter in a saucepan.

- Boil with continuous stirring.

- Afterwards, stir in the garlic.

- Remove from stovetop.

- Whisk the eggs and then pour it into the broth.

- Stir.

- Leave for a minute to allow the egg to cook.

- Enjoy your warm meal!

17) Keto Mustard Pork Loins

4 pcs. 114 g pork loins

4 oz. organic chicken broth

2 oz. full-fat cream

1 tsp. organic apple cider vinegar

1 tbsp. sea salt

1 tbsp. mustard

1 tsp. paprika

1 tbsp. lemon

1 tsp. thyme

1 tsp. black pepper, freshly ground

- Use paper towels to pat the meat dry.

- Then, rub salt, pepper, thyme, and paprika on both sides.

- Adjust the stove's setting to high heat.

- Sear the meat on each side for a couple of minutes.

- Pour the chicken broth into the same skillet.

- Next, add the full-fat cream and the apple cider vinegar. Simmer.

- Pour in the lemon juice.

- Stir in the mustard.

- Afterwards, put the pork chops back into the skillet.

- Make sure that both sides are well-coated.

- Cook for approximately ten minutes with the pan's lid partially open.

18) Keto Cobb Salad

56 g chicken breast, cooked and shredded

128 g spinach, torn to bite-sized pieces

¼ avocado, cubed

1 egg, free-range and hard-boiled and sliced

2 slices bacon, cooked and chopped

½ tomato, sliced

½ tsp. extra virgin olive oil

½ tsp. white vinegar

- Mix the oil and the vinegar.

- Place all the ingredients in a salad bowl.

- Toss well and eat up!

19) Keto Chicken Parm

1 egg, free-range

450 g. chicken breast

28 g pork rinds

4 oz. mozzarella, shredded

2 tbsp. parmesan

4 oz. marinara sauce

Sea salt

Freshly ground black pepper

Desired amount of garlic powder

Desired amount of oregano

- First, warm up the oven to 350 F.

- In a food processor, combine the parmesan and the pork rinds. Pulse until both are well-crushed and you get a breading-like mixture.

- Transfer the processor's contents into a plate.

- Lay the chicken breasts on a clean flat surface.

- Cover the meat with some plastic wrap.

- Pound the meat until they are a half inch thin. Make sure that the chicken has been flattened uniformly to ensure even cooking of the meat.

- Whisk the eggs.

- Dip the chicken breasts into the eggs.

- Afterwards, press the meat into the breading mixture, ensuring that all sides are evenly coated.

- Grease a baking pan with some organic butter, coconut oil, or cooking spray.

- Arrange the meat on the baking dish and sprinkle with desired amounts of salt, pepper, garlic, and oregano.

- Place the dish in the oven and cook for approximately 23-26 minutes. The crust should have a nice golden brown hue.

- Remove the dish from the oven.

- Pour marinara sauce over the meat.

- Add the mozzarella on top.

- Then, return the dish into the oven and cook for another 13-16 minutes.

20) Ketogenic Pesto and Feta Omelet

3 eggs, free-range

1 tbsp. organic butter

1 oz. feta cheese

1 tbsp. full-fat cream

1 tbsp. pesto

Sea salt

Black pepper, freshly ground

- In a skillet, melt the butter.

- Whisk the eggs together with the full-fat cream.

- Pour the eggs into the hot skillet.

- When the eggs are almost cooked, add the feta cheese on one side of the omelet. Then, slather pesto all over the feta cheese.

- Fold your omelet.

- Continue cooking for four more minutes to allow the cheese to melt.

21) Keto Halloumi Salad

1 cucumber, sliced

250 g baby arugula, sliced

85 g. halloumi cheese, sliced to 1/3-inch pieces

141 g walnuts, chopped

7 cherry tomatoes

Extra virgin olive oil

Balsamic vinegar

Sea salt

- First, grill the halloumi cheese. 4 minutes on each side should do the trick.

- Combine the arugula, the cherry tomatoes, and the cucumber in a bowl.

- Add the chopped walnuts. Toss well.

- Sprinkle desired amount of salt.

- Drizzle with oil and vinegar.

- Dig in!

22) Ketogenic Quarter Pounders

226 g beef, ground

1 egg, free-range, beaten

1 slice bacon, finely chopped

2 tbsp. organic butter

1 tbsp. jalapenos, finely sliced

2 leaves iceberg lettuce

1 tbsp. organic mayonnaise

½ tsp. sea salt

¼ onion, sliced

½ tsp. red pepper flakes

1 tsp. sriracha

½ tsp. basil, finely chopped

½ tomato, diced

¼ tsp. cayenne

- Knead the ground meat for a couple of minutes.

- Combine the tomato, the bacon, the jalapenos, the egg, the sriracha and the other spices with the meat.

- Take a few minutes to knead the meat well to ensure even distribution of the ingredients.

- Divide the meat into four equal portions. Using your palms, make four patties.

- Add a tablespoonful of butter on each of two patties.

- Afterwards, lay the non-buttered patties on top of the buttered ones.

- Seal the sides well. This way, you'll have two butter-filled patties.

- Cook on an open grill. After 5 minutes, flip the patties.

- Add the onion slices to caramelize them. After 2 ½ minutes, flip the onions.

- Arrange the iceberg lettuce on two serving plates. Slater some mayo on each lettuce.

- Lay the patties on your green "buns" and top with caramelized onions.

- Sink your teeth into this tasty lunch!

23) Classic Keto Tuna Salad

2 eggs, free-range, hard-boiled and sliced

100 g romaine lettuce, washed and torn

140 g tuna, boiled

2 tbsp. homemade mayonnaise

15 g chives, chopped

Juice from ½ lemon

1 tbsp. extra virgin olive oil

Sea salt

- Arrange the lettuce in a bowl.

- Add the tuna and egg slices.

- Spoon some mayonnaise and squeeze some lemon juice. Toss.

- Top with chives.

- Lastly, drizzle with olive oil.

24) Keto Gnochi

3 egg yolks, free-range

16 oz. mozzarella, shredded

2 tbsp. coconut oil

1 tsp. sea salt

1 tsp. garlic, minced

- In the oven toaster, melt the mozzarella. Do this for ten minutes. Stir from time to time.

- Whisk the yolks with the garlic and the salt. Then, pour the mixture over the melted mozzarella. Mix well.

- Divide the mixture into four. Roll on a parchment paper to create four long and slender strips.

- Chop the strips to 1 inch slices to make your gnocchi.

- Boil a potful of water.

- One by one, drop the gnocchi.

- Eventually, they will float in the water. When this happens, drain water.

- Afterwards, fry the gnocchi in a skillet with coconut oil.

- Buon appètito!

25) Keto Rosemary Chicken

4 pcs. organic chicken thighs

4 fresh rosemary sprigs

Juice from 1/2 lemon

½ lemon, quartered

2 tbsp. organic butter

Sea salt

Freshly ground black pepper

1 garlic clove, chopped

- First, warm up the oven to 400 F.

- Adjust the stove's setting to high. Preheat a cast iron skillet.

- Rub salt and pepper evenly on all sides of the meat.

- Once the pan is hot, sear the chicken for 5 minutes. Make sure that the skin side is in contact with the pan.

- Afterwards, flip the thighs over.

- Add lemon juice on the skin side of the chicken.

- Throw in the quartered lemon into the skillet.

- Add the garlic and rosemary.

- Next, place the pan in the oven.

- Baking time is ½ hour.

- Remove the pan from the oven and slather some butter on the chicken.

- Again, place the pan in the oven and cook for an extra 10 minutes.

- Eat well!

Chapter 4:
Fit as a Foodie:
Keto Dinner Recipes

26) Keto Lime Cod

1 egg, free range

10 oz. cod fillets, wild-caught

45 g coconut flour

1 tsp. red pepper, crushed

Juice from 1 lime

1 tsp. sea salt

1 ½ tsp. garlic, minced

½ tsp. cayenne

- Warm up the oven to 400 F.

- Beat the egg.

- Pour the coconut flour into a shallow dish.

- Dip the fish into the egg for about 60 seconds.

- Afterwards, press both sides of the fish into the coco flour.

- Lay the fish on a baking pan.

- Sprinkle red pepper, cayenne, garlic, and salt.

- Add the lime juice, squeezing evenly into each fillet.

- Season and arrange on cooking sheet

- Place the baking pan in the oven. Cooking time is about 11 minutes.

- Enjoy your dinner!

27) Keto Zucchini Aglio e Olio

16 oz. zucchini, shredded

3 tbsp. organic butter, salted

1 tbsp. olive oil

2 oz. parmesan, grated

2 tsp. red pepper, chopped

2 oz. Italian cow's milk cheese, shaved

1 tbsp. garlic, minced

1 tbsp. basil, chopped

Sea salt

Black pepper, freshly cracked

- Adjust the stove's setting to medium heat.

- In a saucepan, melt the butter.

- Add the olive oil.

- Next, throw in the garlic and the red pepper.

- Sauté for about 60 seconds.

- Add the shredded zucchini. Cook for a couple of minutes.

- Remove from stovetop.

- Add the parmesan and the basil. Toss.

- Transfer into a serving bowl.

- Use the cheese as toppings.

28) Keto Simple Pot Roast

96 oz. roast-sized beef

16 oz. beef broth

2 tbsp. dehydrated parsley

1 tbsp. buttermilk powder

¼ tsp. thyme

2 tbsp. garlic powder

½ tsp. basil

1 ½ tsp. dehydrated dill weed

¼ tsp. celery powder

2 tbsp. freshly ground black pepper

1 tbsp. oregano, chopped

2 tbsp. onion powder

- Place the beef in the slow cooker along with the broth.
- Mix the rest of the ingredients in a large bowl. Combine thoroughly and store in an airtight jar.
- Take 1 tbsp. of the mixture and add 6 tbsp. into the pot roast.
- Cook in the slow cooker in low setting for approximately 8 hours.
- Guten appètit!

29) Brussels Sprouts Salad

6 Brussels sprouts, washed, cut thinly lengthways and roots removed

½ tsp. organic apple cider vinegar

1 tbsp. parmesan, grated

1 tsp. grape seed oil

Sea salt

Freshly ground black pepper

- Place the sprouts in a bowl.

- Drizzle apple cider vinegar and grape seed oil.

- Add desired amount of salt and pepper.

- Use parmesan as toppings.

- Toss well and enjoy!

30) Keto Sweet Pea Coco Hash

7 oz. pea pods, stringless, chopped

4 tbsp. organic butter, salted

4 oz. coconut, shredded

1 tbsp. olive oil

1/8 tsp. cinnamon

1 tbsp. fresh rosemary

Sea salt

- Adjust the stove's setting to medium-low.

- In a skillet, melt the butter and then add the olive oil.

- Add the shredded coconut and stir well.

- Throw in the rosemary.

- Add the cinnamon and mix well.

- Adjust the stove's setting to low heat. Continue cooking for about 60 seconds.

- Incorporate the pea pods.

- Increase the heat to medium and cook for 4-6 minutes.

- Sprinkle desired amount of salt.

31) Quick Steak and Cheese

16 oz. shaved steak

4 slices medium-firm and salty-sweet cheese

1 tbsp. ghee

2 tbsp. homemade mayonnaise

32 g onions, chopped

32 g bell peppers, chopped

1 tbsp. coconut oil

1 tbsp. Dijon mustard

1 tbsp. garlic, minced

- Adjust the stove's setting to medium low.

- In a pan, melt the ghee.

- Then, sauté the onions, the garlic, and the bell peppers until they yield a fragrant aroma.

- Pour the coconut oil into the skillet.

- Next, throw in the steak. Cook the meat until perfectly browned.

- Adjust the stove's setting to low.

- Stir in the mayonnaise and the mustard. Mix well.

- Top the meat with cheese. Leave for about one minute to allow the cheese to melt.

- Once the cheese has melted, mix well and serve.

32) Magical Meat Muffins

6 egg yolks, free-range

450 g beef, ground

8 oz. mushrooms

96 g coconut flour

2 tbsp. coco aminos

1 tsp. sea salt

- First, heat up the oven to 350 F.

- Place the mushrooms and the egg yolks in a food processor.

- Add the salt and the coco aminos.

- Pulse until you obtain a nice puree.

- Pour the puree into a bowl.

- Combine the mixture well with the ground beef.

- Using a sifter add the coconut flour into the mixture.

- Now that you have your dough, form small balls using your hands.

- Distribute each meatball into prepared muffin cups.

- Place the muffin tins in the oven. Baking time is around 45 minutes. The outside should be brown while the inside must be moist.

33) Chicken Liver Pate on Radish

1 radish, sliced

100 g chicken liver

3 tbsp. organic butter, softened

½ tsp. sage

½ tsp. thyme

Black pepper, freshly ground

A pinch of sea salt

- Sauté the liver. Leave to cool.

- Combine the liver and the rest of the ingredients in a food processor.

- Pulse until you get a nice smooth paste.

- Spread the pate on the radish slices and enjoy munching on your light dinner!

34) Keto Zucchini Noodle Soup

48 oz. organic chicken broth

450 g organic chicken breast, thinly sliced

1 zucchini, shredded

1 tbsp. olive oil

15 oz. coconut milk

2 tbsp. curry paste

2 garlic cloves, minced

2 tbsp. fish sauce

½ white onion, chopped

1 lime, wedged

64 g cilantro, chopped

1 red pepper, cut thinly

½ jalapeno, sliced

- Adjust the stove's setting to medium.

- Heat the olive oil in a saucepan. Sauté the onions for approximately 5 minutes.

- Add the curry paste and the jalapeno. Throw in the garlic. Cook with constant stirring for about 60 seconds.

- With brisk whisking, pour in the broth and the milk. Increase the stove's setting to high.

- Once the broth begins to boil, lower the stove's setting to medium.

- Include the chicken.

- Then, add the red pepper slices and the fish sauce.

- Simmer for 5 minutes.

- Afterwards, you may add the cilantro. Stir well.

- Distribute the zucchini evenly into 8 serving bowls.

- Pour the hot soup over the zucchini. This will tenderize the "noodles".

- Serve with a slice of lime on the side.

Note: This recipe serves 8 guests.

35) Keto Steak and Chimichurri

155 g sirloin steak

A bunch of parsley, chopped

16 oz. romaine lettuce, torn

2 cloves garlic

2 radishes, cut thinly

2 tbsp. lemon juice

43 g red cabbage, torn

½ tsp. chili flakes

2 ½ tbs. olive oil

1 shallot, chopped

2 tbsp. cilantro, chopped

2 tsp. red wine vinegar

½ tsp. oregano

Sea salt

Freshly ground black pepper

- Begin by making the chimichurri sauce. In a food processor, combine the shallot, the garlic, the parsley, the chili flakes, and the oregano.

- Pour in 2 tbsp. of the olive oil. Add 1 tbsp. lemon juice and the vinegar. If you wish, add desired amount of salt and pepper. Pulse until you get a nice rich yet smooth consistency.

- Use the remaining ½ tbsp. olive oil and slather it all over the meat. Rub salt and pepper on the steaks.

- Combine the cabbage, the lettuce, the radish, and the cilantro in a bowl. Drizzle with the remaining 1 tbsp. lemon.

- Cook the steaks on an open grill. A couple of minutes on each side should do the trick.

- Serve the steak with the sauce and salad.

36) Keto Chicken Chowder

450 g organic chicken thighs, deboned and skin removed

8 oz. chicken broth, organic

16 oz. tomatoes, diced

8 oz. cream cheese

1 shallot, chopped

1 jalapeno, chopped

2 tbsp. lime juice

1 garlic clove, chopped

1 tsp. sea salt

1 tbsp. black pepper, freshly ground

- Place all the ingredients in a crock pot.

- Adjust the setting to high.

- Cook for approximately 4 hours.

- When the meat is ready, use forks to shred the chicken.

- Enjoy eating!

37) Keto Caesar Salad

4 pcs. anchovy fillets

24 leaves romaine lettuce, washed

8 tbsp. parmesan, grated

2 oz. pork rinds, crushed

1 tsp. homemade mayonnaise

2 cloves garlic

- In a blender, combine the mayonnaise and the anchovies.

- Incorporate the parmesan and the garlic.

- Blend using the lowest setting.

- Now that you have your dressing, distribute the lettuce evenly among 4 salad dishes.

- Drizzle the mixture into the lettuce.

- Use the pork rinds in lieu of carb-rich croutons.

- Top with more shredded parmesan.

38) Keto Chicken Skewers

680 g chicken tenderloin

½ tbsp. olive oil

½ tsp. sea salt

½ tsp. freshly ground black pepper

Fresh thyme sprigs

10 pcs. wooden skewers

- Soak the skewers in cold water.

- Warm up the oven to 350 F.

- In a bowl, combine the chicken meat with the rest of the ingredients.

- Pierce the meat with the wooden sticks.

- Arrange on a baking dish and cook for about 40 minutes.

- Enjoy your dinner!

Chapter 5:
Smart, Sexy Snacks

39) Keto Cheese Balls

4 oz. goat cheese

4 oz. pistachios, shells removed and crushed

Sea salt

- Divide the goat cheese into seven slices.

- With your hands, make balls with the slices.

- Combine the pistachios with desired amount of sea salt.

- Then, roll the cheese balls into the crushed nuts. Make sure that all sides are well-covered.

- Go on, go crazy!

40) Keto Stuffed Eggs

6 eggs, free-range

128 g organic chicken, boiled and shredded

2 tbsp. homemade mayonnaise

1 tbsp. shallots, chopped

½ tsp. dill

1 tbsp. Dijon mustard

½ tsp. freshly ground black pepper

Sea salt

- In a bowl, combine all the ingredients with the exception of the eggs.

- Place in the fridge.

- When the salad is cold, you can start boiling the eggs.

- Remove the shell and cut into halves. Carefully scoop out the yolks.

- Spoon the salad to fill the hollow in each egg.

- Sprinkle with a seasoning powder of your choice. Spanish paprika powder is recommended.

41) Strawberry Cheesecake Smoothie

4 oz. strawberries

8 oz. almond milk

1 oz. cream cheese

1 tbsp. vanilla syrup (no sugar)

- Combine all these ingredients in a blender.

- Blend until you obtain a smooth texture.

- Bottoms up!

42) Quick Dill Pickle Tuna Sandwich

3 oz. tuna flakes

3 tbsp. homemade mayonnaise

Dill pickles, sliced lengthways

Sea salt

Freshly ground black pepper

- With the exception of the pickles, mix all the ingredients in a bowl.

- Keep in the refrigerator overnight.

- Next, slather the tuna mixture all over the slices of dill.

- Enjoy!

43) Strawberry Zucchini Noodle Salad

8 oz. zucchini, shredded

8 oz. strawberries, sliced

2 tbsp. balsamic vinegar

1 tbsp. goat cheese, sliced and crushed

2 tbsp. olive oil

1 tbsp. pistachios

1/8 tsp. sea salt

1/8 tsp. pepper, freshly cracked

½ tsp. garlic, minced

- Combine the zucchini, the goat cheese, and the nuts in a bowl. Toss.

- Take half of the strawberries and arrange them over the salad.

- Mix the rest of the strawberries, the vinegar, and the oil in a blender.

- Add garlic. Sprinkle sea salt and pepper.

- Blend well.

- Transfer the dressing into a glass container. This is to be refrigerated.

- If you're in a rush, take 1 tbsp. of the dressing and drizzle it on top of your salad.

Note: The recipe for the dressing is good for 4 salads.

44) Egg Cream Keto Shake

2 eggs, free-range

2 oz. full-fat cream

2 tbsp. cream cheese

2 tbsp. raw wild honey to sweeten

4 pcs. ice cubes

- Throw all the ingredients together in a blender.

- Process until you get a creamy consistency.

- Enjoy your quick drink!

45) Coco Berry Smoothie

8 oz. coconut milk, unsweetened

6 pcs. fresh strawberries

4 tbsp. full-fat cream

2 tbsp. raw wild honey

- Place all the ingredients in a blender.

- Blend well until perfectly smooth.

- Take your snack in the kitchen or to go!

46) Ketogenic Truffles

8 oz. peanut butter, chunky

5 tbsp. coconut butter

Desiccated coconut

16 oz. full-fat cream

- Prepare a muffin tray by spraying each cup with cooking spray.

- In a blender, combine the peanut butter and the cream.

- Pour the mixture into a Ziploc bag.

- Include the coconut butter. Seal.

- Massage the bag with your hands until the ingredients are thoroughly combined.

- At the bottom corner of the plastic bag, make a half-inch cut. This way, you have an improvised pipette.

- Squeeze to fill each muffin cup at about ¾ full.

- Place in the freezer for at least half an hour before indulging.

Note: This recipe makes up to 30 truffles.

47) Keto Choco-Orange Drink

1 handful spinach

8 oz. cashew milk

2 scoops whey protein powder (chocolate flavored)

1 tbsp. pure orange juice

6 pcs. ice cubes

- In a blender, combine all of the ingredients.

- Process until you are able to make a smooth and creamy drink.

- Pour into a tall glass and enjoy!

48) Garlicky Keto Edamame

10 oz. frozen edamame, steamed

2 tbsp. olive oil

2 oz. parmesan, grated

1 tsp. red pepper flakes

1 tsp. garlic, minced

- Heat the oil in a skillet.

- Throw in the garlic and the pepper flakes.

- Adjusting the stove to low setting, sauté until the garlic is almost browned.

- Remove from stovetop.

- Add the edamame into the skillet and toss well.

- In a serving bowl, mix the edamame with the parmesan.

- Enjoy!

49) Ketogenic Peanut Butter Cups

1 stick organic butter, unsalted

4 tbsp. peanut butter

67 g sugar alternative, granulated

1 oz. dark chocolate, unsweetened

2 tbsp. full-fat cream

Walnuts, chopped

- In a saucepan, quickly melt the chocolate and the butter in high heat with continuous stirring.

- Pour in the sweetener. Mix thoroughly.

- Next, add the peanut butter.

- Pour in the cream. Stir well.

- Use parchment paper to line the muffin cups.

- Then, arrange the chopped nuts at the bottom of each cup

- Scoop the mixture into each cup until they're ¾ full.

- Place in the freezer for approximately 1 hour or until the peanut butter cups become firm.

- Feel free to indulge without the guilt!

50) Salted Caramel Keto Smoothie

8 oz. cashew milk

3 tbsp. full-fat cream

2 tbsp. caramel syrup (no sugar)

6 pcs. ice cubes

A dash of pumpkin pie spice

- Mix all the ingredients into your trusty blender.

- Blend until you get a smooth-textured mixture.

- Pour into a serving glass and drink to your health!

Conclusion

Thank you again for purchasing this book!

I hope this book was able to help you experience an epicurean expedition which leads to one great destination: the fulfillment of your ultimate fitness goal.

The next step is to explore these recipes for wellness and to start cooking (and eating!) your way to a sexier, healthier new you.

Thank you and good luck!

Made in the USA
San Bernardino, CA
20 May 2018